Open to Change:
The Power of Reflection in Your Yoga Practice

Open to Change:
The Power of Reflection in Your Yoga Practice

FRAN BRUNKE

iUniverse, Inc.
New York   Bloomington

Copyright © 2009 Fran Brunke

All rights reserved. No part of this book may be used or reproduced by any means, graphic, electronic, or mechanical, including photocopying, recording, taping or by any information storage retrieval system without the written permission of the publisher except in the case of brief quotations embodied in critical articles and reviews.

iUniverse books may be ordered through booksellers or by contacting:

iUniverse
1663 Liberty Drive
Bloomington, IN 47403
www.iuniverse.com
1-800-Authors (1-800-288-4677)

Because of the dynamic nature of the Internet, any Web addresses or links contained in this book may have changed since publication and may no longer be valid. The views expressed in this work are solely those of the author and do not necessarily reflect the views of the publisher, and the publisher hereby disclaims any responsibility for them.

ISBN: 978-1-4401-4797-5 (sc)
ISBN: 978-1-4401-4798-2 (ebook)

Printed in the United States of America

iUniverse rev. date: 10/5/2009

Also by Fran Brunke:

Sol: Salutations to the Sun CD

"I maintain that Truth is a pathless land, and you cannot approach it by any path whatsoever, by any religion, by any sect."

J. Krishnamurti

Contents

Acknowledgments	xiii
Introduction	xv
Being Open to Change	xvi
More Than "Just" Physical Practice	xvii
Change and the Family of Humanity	xviii

Chapter 1: Evolving Your Mature Practice

Cultivating Beginner's Mind	1
Instead of Doing the Pose, Be the Pose	2
Reflect: Download and Record Impressions	4
How Long Does It Take?	5
What about My Current Practice?	7
How to Do the Reflections	7
A Word about Nonharming (*Ahimsa*)	9
What to Do While Being the Pose	9

Chapter 2: Standing Poses

Contemplation: Please Remove Shoes Before Entering	13
Mountain Pose	16
Half-Moon Pose	19
Triangle Pose	21
Warrior 1, Warrior 2	24

Chapter 3: Standing Balance Poses

Contemplation: Facing the Desire for Perfection	29

Tree Pose	31
Balancing Warrior Pose (Warrior 3)	34

Chapter 4: Belly-Lying Poses

Contemplation: Healing on All Levels	37
Energy Signature in Belly-Lying Poses	39
Deepening Your Experience with Sound	39
Sphinx Pose	41
Cobra Pose	44
Boat Pose	46
Bow Pose	49

Chapter 5: Three Poses from Hands and Knees (Table Position)

Downward-Facing Dog Pose	53
Belly Awareness in Downward-Facing Dog	55
Pigeon Pose	58
Child's Pose	61

Chapter 6: Forward Bends

Contemplation: The Symbolism of Forward Bends	65
Hero Pose	67
Hero Pose with Forward Bend	69
Head-to-Knee Pose	70
Seated Forward Bend	72

Chapter 7: Twists

Contemplation: The Dark Side of Twists	75

Half-Lord of the Fishes Pose	77
Reclined Spinal Twist	80

Chapter 8: Supine Poses

Contemplation: Working with Gravity	83
Bridge Pose	85
Fish Pose	88
Plow Pose	90

Conclusion	95

Acknowledgments

I wish to acknowledge and honor here all traditions and lineages of yoga. I am especially grateful to the Kripalu teachings and tradition because that is where I found my spiritual awakening. To Bille von Roeder, who was my first real teacher, and all the many beautiful teachers and shining spirits it has been my good fortune to learn from at Kripalu Center, and to all who came before them, *jai bhagwan.*

Thanks to Mark McNeely, who brought the beautiful brushstroke images into reality.

To Karla Jacobsen, owner and founder of Blue Door Yoga Room for her vision, constant support, and encouragement; and Mary DelleDonne, for her intuition, faith, and goddess card readings.

To my husband, supporter, and soul mate Denis, who became a yogi in his own way and in his own time.

To the beautiful souls in the Blue Door Yoga Room community who had faith, showed up, and contributed: this book would not have been possible without your divine support.

To Velta and Doug Bush for the best possible writing environment a person could wish for.

And to all students, past, present, and future: *tat tvam asi.*

Namaste,
Fran Brunke
Playa Hermosa, Costa Rica
March 2009

Introduction

The many various yoga traditions are gateways or portals that can lead to understanding our own truth. For each of us, the truth will be something unique, something infinite, and possibly something beyond tradition.

I used to believe that there was always a "right" answer or correct destination, that by doing good yoga I would get somewhere, and that place would be the right place. I look back fondly on that belief as if I were a cute little toddler learning to walk.

My work as a yoga teacher has taken me to a new understanding. First, it has made me more open to change. I understand now that all questions have many "right" answers, depending on the levels of meaning being addressed. Second, I've also come to believe that there are many "right" ways to do any pose.

Learning begins with being told what's right and

then doing that. The authentic learning comes later, through self-discovery: what feels right now, what alignment works best at this particular time, and what lights us up in the present moment. While there are many "right" ways to do a pose, there is only one way to *be* the pose, and that is to hold the pose long enough, without any attachment whatsoever to correctness, perfection, or end result.

For all of us, that is where the real truth lies because that is where the true self waits—in the present moment.

Being Open to Change

This book is designed to give you a method for self-inquiry that will help you evolve personally as your yoga practice evolves. Or vice versa—it may help you evolve your practice and, so to speak, catch up to your new, evolving self. It's for practitioners who already have a regular yoga practice in place and who are ready to deepen that practice. I assume here that you already know how to do the poses and that you understand the precautions and contraindications. Nothing in this book can replace the need for a good teacher, nor can it launch a beginner practice.

More Than "Just" Physical Practice

Yoga is much more than "just" physical: yoga is extra-physical from the first breath. From the first attempt at Tadasana to the most fluid Surya Namaskar, the body is the gateway into an ever-deepening connection between your mind, your emotions, and your inner self. It's been my experience that it can take at least a few years of practice to discover this extra-physical aspect.

The poses in this book are not terrifically advanced. In fact, they are twenty-two of the most no-frills foundation poses. But here, they are practiced at a more advanced level. Many excellent books, CDs, and videos are now available to be consulted as instructional guides, so I make no attempt to teach you how to do the poses or master them. The reflective approach to practice in this book is best suited for those who have already been practicing yoga for at least a couple of years.

In mainstream North American yoga culture, it has become unfashionable to practice the foundation poses. We want to advance quickly. We want to be promoted to the higher grades without delay. Like everything else, even in yoga, we push ourselves so we can do more, do it in less time, and do it more efficiently. We want to get there now, please—right away if at all possible.

This approach can leave us profoundly disconnected and unhappy in life and in yoga.

Furthermore, it can lead us away from what we were looking for in yoga in the first place. If you are looking for speed, action, and gymnastics, this is not the book for you.

The message in this book is this:
- The body's way of talking to you is through how you feel.
- Therefore, how you feel is important.
- Reflecting upon what you feel will lead you to self-knowledge.
- In self-knowledge lies your truth.

Change and the Family of Humanity

Sages have told us that the whole goal of yoga is self-knowledge. For most of us, though, yoga begins as a physical endeavor. Through the gateway of the body, practiced regularly and over a long period of time, yoga will inevitably take you into your feelings and your thoughts. Through knowing these thoughts and feelings better, you become much more discerning and powerful. In other words, your awareness of your self increases through dedicated practice.

As awareness increases, yoga will take you to where the mind and the body interconnect. At this level, yoga can help you shed old patterns, habits, and camouflage of all sorts. You can meet yourself where you are, and that is a very good place, much as you may mistrust it because it is so filled with change.

The body has its own language and will always tell you the truth. Asana gives us the perfect environment in which to listen to those messages. The only trouble is that the messages are in code. Therefore, to listen well to one's own body is an art.

Through the approach in this book, you can deepen your own personal yoga practice. You can become more conscious, more deliberate, and more powerful. You can uncover yourself gradually, layer by layer.

And what is revealed will be surprising to you. You will come to know that what is inside you is human, yes, but that beyond that, you are something more. You may just become more acceptable to yourself, more loving toward yourself, and more aware of your worth. It is my hope that you will come to know, without a doubt, that at your core, you are truly remarkable, powerful, and blessed.

From my point of view, this is how yoga serves the family of humanity in the current times of great change. When individuals can appreciate themselves for who they really are and what they really are, then we can fully appreciate other people for who they are, too—not for who they want to be or wish to be. When we are open to changing how we think of ourselves, then we set ourselves free to experience life differently.

At this point in my life and teaching career, it seems obvious that world peace actually begins with being at peace with oneself. That represents a huge change for most of us, even people who have practiced yoga for some years. There will be some who argue against it or dismiss it out of hand—so be it. All I can tell is my truth. May it be your truth, too.

Chapter 1

Evolving Your Mature Practice

One way to advance your practice is, of course, to practice more challenging poses. Another way is to practice simple poses with a more advanced attitude. For this approach to work, your body needs previous yoga experience, while what is required mentally is a certain humility to show up as if you know nothing at all.

In simple terms, the method proposed here is meant to deepen your practice and understand the code of your body's language. I am suggesting three key strategies.

1. Cultivating Beginner's Mind

Practicing simple poses in an advanced way requires a new mind-set. Additionally, it requires a radical reversal of what is usually intended by the word "advanced."

You do already know how to do these poses with real competence and skill. In addition, you are likely acquainted with the more physically challenging, and therefore more interesting, poses. Perhaps the bigger the physical challenge is, the more interested you are in doing the pose. Beginner's mind requires that you leave that aside, just for the moment. Can you temporarily clear your own hard-won knowledge and experience from your mind? Are you willing to include one humble foundation pose in your practice and do it as if you knew nothing about it? Can you approach it as if there were nothing in your memory bank about it?

To move away from the assumption that you already know all this stuff takes you into new territory. Just to be present with a simple old friend such as Mountain Pose in this way requires us to set aside any notion of having been there before or of knowing what to expect. This is what Buddhist friends might call beginner's mind.

2. Instead of *Doing* the Pose, *Be* the Pose

Second, choose one simple pose as the

"focus pose" in your yoga practice that day. Stay in that pose long enough to allow the body to speak. If you stay with it long enough, at some point, you will no longer be "doing" the pose; you will *be* the pose itself. At that moment, there is no separation between you, your body, and your pose. When that happens, there is an element of timelessness, and if you are practicing in a receptive way, you will receive information. Sometimes that information may take shape as an insight or as spontaneous integration. At other times, it may be less precise.

Every time you do a pose, it's as if you are signing your name to it. It becomes uniquely yours. At the same time, the pose is signing itself onto you, too. It is becoming known to you by making its mark on your energy as well as on your body.

It starts with the alignment and the doing, but ultimately, the signature of the pose is in the energy of it. The energy of the pose is something that goes beyond details of alignment. The brushstroke illustrations in this book are intended to help you focus on the energy rather than the precise anatomical details.

3. Reflect: Download and Record Impressions

The third key is to download the impressions and sensations you receive. That's where the journaling comes in. The body will never lie to you. By writing about your experience shortly after you practice, you can clarify the feelings, bits of awareness, or thoughts that came to you. It is a simple method through which you can access your own truth from a deep, eternal place.

Journaling has long been a part of my personal practice. For as long as I have been practicing yoga, I have been journaling. In a sense, I think of myself as a journalist—not for a newspaper, but for myself. Journaling has helped me stay in touch with my own changes. The nature of my practice is very different now than it was when I started thirty years ago. As I have changed, so has my yoga practice. Those changes used to worry me, but now I see a natural evolution. Both yoga and journaling have helped me stay aligned with my own truth through all the changes.

Journaling does the same thing as looking in the mirror. The writing in your journal gives you a mirror into your spirit and your personal truth. It's a powerful tool for seeing into the nonphysical (or extraphysical) aspect of your yoga.

To say this another way, the writing allows you to listen to and understand your higher self. By journaling, you will crack your own code. You will become more conscious, more deliberate, and more powerful. You will reveal your true self gradually, layer by layer.

How Long Does It Take?

This may be the quintessential North American question. The dictates of modern studio practice are such that longer holdings are not encouraged. While there's time to "do" the poses, there may be no time to "be" the pose. There's no time to be timeless. But timelessness is where the magic lies. This is the gift you can give yourself in your home practice.

It takes a while to realize that yoga practice is something more than or other than a physical practice. Some people know right away; others will make the discovery in their own time. It's the same with practicing your focus pose for the day: there is no definition of how long "a while" will be. Only you can decide.

The length of time for a focus pose is not a specific number of breaths, but it will probably be more breaths than you would usually allow for one pose. It's not a specific number of seconds or minutes, either. If you stay long enough, with an open and curious attitude, you will be outside of time. If you stay long enough in the pose, steadily, breathing smoothly, and quiet inside, you will access the timeless nature that is available to us when we practice yoga.

Put the focus pose somewhere in the middle of your routine, or let it be the final pose you do that day. What works best for me is to make it the last or almost-last pose. After coming out of the focus pose, I sit with my journal. I don't try to analyze; I just write what comes without editing or judging. It's like a little meditation in writing. Then I put down my pen and go into savasana.

Plan your focus pose in advance, or just let yourself decide spontaneously in the moment. You can pick any pose on any day. It would be equally useful to skip around for variety or to stay with one particular focus pose for a few days or weeks.

Let your intuition guide you. You cannot get it wrong. Whatever your regular practice looks like, just allow some time for one focus pose and then do a little journaling.

What about My Current Practice?

You don't need to change your practice. It's established, it works for you—let it be. For instance, if you have a strong Ashtanga practice, there is no need to change that. What I am encouraging you to do is to continue with a slightly different focus. First, make space in your mind for beginner's mind, and then make space in your practice for one focus posture and a little time for your journal. That's it.

How to Do the Reflections

Simply do your practice, and as soon as you can after the focus pose, preferably before final relaxation, write whatever comes to you. Some days there will be lots to write; sometimes there won't be very much. Don't worry about it.

Express yourself clearly and quickly. If you can't find the right words, then draw a picture and label it. It can be totally liberating to use color—markers, gel pens, and highlighters. Take a look at any book by Sark to see some glorious, colorful examples. There's also a technique called mind mapping, which involves writing down keywords and some spontaneous associated concepts. Whatever you do, do not worry about grammar or spelling. It needs to be understandable only to you. No one else is meant to read it. Then forget about it. It is what it is. Get on with the rest of your day.

There are many ways to get started with the "what to write" part. You could use any of the ideas expressed in the book as a jumping-off point for your journaling. It will also work if you skip the essays entirely and just write.

A truly simple and effective way to begin is by writing "I want to tell you that..." and then keep going. The "you" being addressed is a kind of benevolent observer, someone who is on your side and to whom you can say anything. This wonderful technique was taught at Kripalu in group sharing workshops, and I have found it to be the quickest, most effective and direct way to begin journaling.

You cannot do this the "wrong way"; please go about it in your own way, be creative, and just trust that it will work. It will work.

Eventually, all the pieces in your journal will add up to something interesting and illuminating, and you will know that it was worth the time and effort.

A Word about Nonharming (*Ahimsa*)

It goes without saying, I hope, that nothing suggested here should cause you physical pain.

Pain is a harsh teacher. Thankfully, there are so many other effective ways of learning. It's worth remembering that the foundation of asana practice is the principle of *ahimsa* (nonharming). If we are creating injuries for ourselves, then we are straying very far from the path. If your focus pose is causing you physical pain, then you have crossed the line and entered the territory of learning through self-harm.

There are contraindications for every pose. There are also modifications for certain physical conditions, including pregnancy. That's why you need a good teacher to get you started correctly.

What to Do While Being the Pose

The following process is a perpetual cycle based on the advice that my Kripalu teachers gave me years ago. It is very simple, and it will lead you into a natural deepening of your practice. *It is more about being aware than about being correct.*

While you're in the pose, there are five things for you to be doing:
1. Breathing
2. Relaxing
3. Feeling
4. Listening
5. Allowing

Breathe: Every pose starts and ends with the breath. Breathe in and out through the nose. Just start with the intention of keeping your breath smooth and steady, and then keep it smooth and steady. Use *dirgha* or *ujjayi* breathing. Keep checking in on your breathing. If it becomes ragged or if you find yourself holding your breath, then mindfully do what you need to do to bring it back to a smooth, steady flow.

Relax: It takes concentration to do this. While some muscular tension is necessary in any pose, the quality needs to be balanced and mindful. What you are looking for are the areas where you are holding on for dear life, as if letting go would result in falling off a cliff. Find in the body an area of too-tight tension, and then gently soften or relax around it. The tension may reappear, or it may become apparent in other locations in the body. Breathe and be aware, softening tight, tense areas as you discover them.

Feel: Once you feel established in the pose and in your breathing, set your attention free to wander inside the framework of the pose. Go into and explore mentally all the corners, angles, and long expanses of the pose. Just notice what's there: what are you feeling in your body and where are you feeling it? What areas feel blank, absent, or restricted? Do not back off from feeling what's really there. Open yourself up to feeling what is presenting itself in the "doing" of the pose.

Listen: What I mean by this is something different from using your ears. It's more like using all the senses. At first, you can hear your breath and your heartbeat. You can discern their unique rhythmic interplay. But in timelessness, true listening will come not from the ears, but rather from the heart. As you do the pose, begin to observe yourself doing the pose. Using all your senses, observe as an impartial observer, not as a Supreme Court justice. Be a witness. Be inside the pose and outside of it simultaneously. Practice open-mindedness. This is where you must release mental tension, if you haven't already. Let go of judging the pose itself. Also relinquish judging yourself in any way. Simply be there, breathing, alert, awake, and open to whatever arises from the domain of physical sensation or from impressions and feelings.

Allow: Another way of saying this is *cultivate*

acceptance. Let yourself be just as you are without accelerating toward anything or pushing anything away. Practice being, not doing. Let yourself be just as you are without needing to change, improve, fix, or compare yourself.

Chapter 2

Standing Poses

Contemplation: Please Remove Shoes Before Entering

There's a sign outside most studio doors: "Please remove your shoes before entering yoga room."

I sometimes think that if there were no sign, people would do the whole yoga practice with their shoes on, even *Savasana.* People don't mean to be disrespectful, necessarily. There is reluctance, especially in new students, to expose our feet. Some people compromise: they wear socks, and it may take six to eight weeks of slipping and sliding before they eventually break down and remove the socks in class.

Do you remember what it's like to walk barefoot on

the sand at the beach, or what it was like to run through cool, soft, grass when you were a kid? Walking barefoot in those conditions just feels good. It's the foot-to-earth contact that feels great.

Part of the reason that it feels so good is that there are important energy centers in the soles of the feet. The soles of the feet are the most absorbent part of the body. If we assume that the earth is itself alive and that we humans are more than simply "passengers" on the planet, then it makes sense that the ground on which we stand would be a constant source of renewable energy coming to us through the feet.

In our modern, concrete world, we've made an art form out of elevating our feet above the ground. Between the soles of our feet and the earth lie layers of concrete, ceramic, tar, rebar, and rubber, which prevent us from ever having to touch the actual earth under our feet. Of course, our feet are protected and they stay cleaner, but we distance ourselves still further from the earth when walking with thick platforms or towering stiletto heels. We spend so little time actually *on* the ground, is it any wonder that many of us feel disconnected and ungrounded these days?

If you ever get the chance to practice yoga outside, you'll be able to experience a whole new dimension to grounding your practice. In the meantime, the yoga mat underneath you represents the earth. In pressing the soles of your feet into the mat, you are connecting metaphorically to the ground of your being. The standing poses that follow are the perfect, most elegant remedy for any ungroundedness or disconnection.

Mountain Pose (*Tadasana*)

Atha yoganusasanam —"Now begins yoga." (Yoga Sutra I.1)

A mountain is deeply connected to and is an integral part of the earth itself. Where does the earth end and the mountain begin? At the same time, the mountain has a point of view that is elevated above earthbound consciousness and concerns.

Mountain Pose is a beautiful metaphor for the human condition. As humans, we possess the same ability to stand deeply rooted and "connected" to life; however, it's also possible to become rather disconnected as if we were mere accidental passengers along for the ride. It's all in how we stand and in our awareness of how we stand.

It takes energy to stand upright. The deployment of that energy is perfectly unique in you. Perhaps you have many different ways of standing. If you change your posture, you thereby change how you show up in any environment. And you change how you relate to other people (or how others relate to you).

Mountain Pose is generally accepted as the foundation for all other standing poses. We can all benefit by standing upright and balanced. Standing tall makes us more aware, more conscious, and more in the picture. We can claim our true power just by practicing any standing poses with attention and focus.

Energy Signature: Mountain Pose (Arms Lifted)

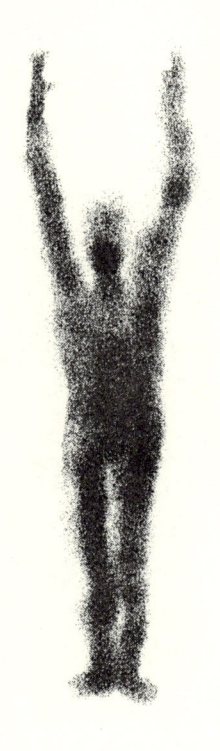

From the outside, the pose may look simple. However, the energy signature here is complex.

Ideally, the body weight will be evenly centered. Inside the framework of the pose, the energy is moving in two directions at once: upward through the feet, legs, spine, and arms; and downward through the arms, spine, legs, and feet.

Half-Moon Pose (*Ardha Chandrasana*)

In its deepest sense, yoga changes us. One of the eternal models of change available to us is the moon. The moon is the fashion diva of the night skies. She never wears the same outfit. She is always changing clothes, always appearing in a new outfit and in a new location.

If the moon were a movie star, an interview with her at the Oscars could never begin with the question, "What's new?" Her answer would be way too complicated; there is always something new with the moon. When is there *not* something new with the moon? The moon is constantly changing, yet in the grand scheme of things, it's also true that the moon is forever the same.

The moon is a reflection of eternity and change at the same time.

What we don't see of the moon is just as important as what we do see. If there were no dark side, then the moon would fall from the sky. There is no struggle to eliminate her dark side; in fact, it is just as important as the bright side. Sometimes, there is more dark than light, but it all comes full circle. As such, the moon gives us a model for healing. Through the illumination of the moon, we can grasp an understanding of what it is like to emerge fully out of our own darkest shadows into our fullness and reveal our true, authentic selves for all to see.

Energy Signature: Half-Moon Pose

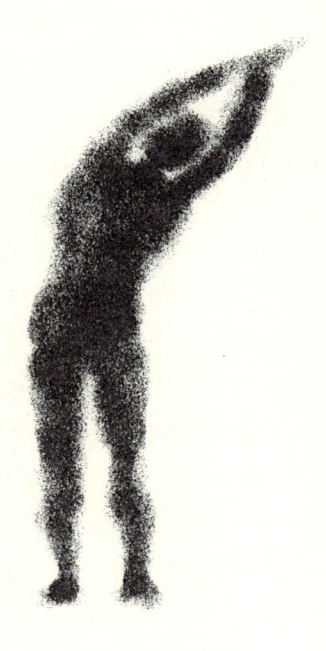

Inside the stillness of this pose, the balance created in Mountain Pose shifts laterally. Notice where the true balance lies. The energy signature here illuminates that healing (becoming whole) must come from integrating that which we choose to reveal with that which desires to remain hidden.

Triangle Pose (*Trikonasana*)

When looking at Triangle Pose for the first time, you can see raw strength, symmetry, and geometry. It's a construction site of a pose, a place where intelligent engineering meets muscle and heavy machinery.

There is no doubt that Triangle Pose requires strength. It is work to be in Triangle, even for a short time. In fact, steel-toed boots would help a lot, especially at the beginning.

But Triangle teaches us to call upon physical strength and turn it into something else—something beyond brute strength, something that is both stronger and lighter than all the muscular strength we may possess.

If practiced with brute force and sheer will to succeed, Triangle Pose will never ripen or open up. Force and aggressiveness will one day boomerang back on us with pain and injury. The magic ingredients are a mix of muscle strength, persistence, and trust. It requires strength and trust to gather all the grounded energy from the legs and the base of the spine and channel it upward to blossom like a flower in the heart. Inside all the geometry of the pose resides a great opening beyond old limits into new parameters. Triangle Pose becomes a gateway for freedom and expansion beyond small-mind limits into a new way of being.

Triangle Pose teaches that the more we can trust in life's support, the lighter life gets.

On the other hand, some of us, men and women alike, are afraid of being perceived as "too strong." Triangle shows us a way to evolve and channel that strength. The more we can appreciate our strength as a gift to be used in the service of opening to our higher purpose, the lighter, freer, and more aligned we become. Triangle shows us how to stay grounded and secure as we branch out into new territory—body, mind, and heart.

To me, Triangle Pose can be seen as the symbol of the global Shift of the Ages: each person grounded in the present moment, stretching out strongly in new directions, and opening up to a more mature understanding of our own individual role in the changes that are upon us now. The one upraised arm provides a perfect pathway from the palm through the centre of the heart right back to Earth. What more elegant metaphor could there be for the New World and for expressing our role in it?

Energy Signature: Triangle Pose

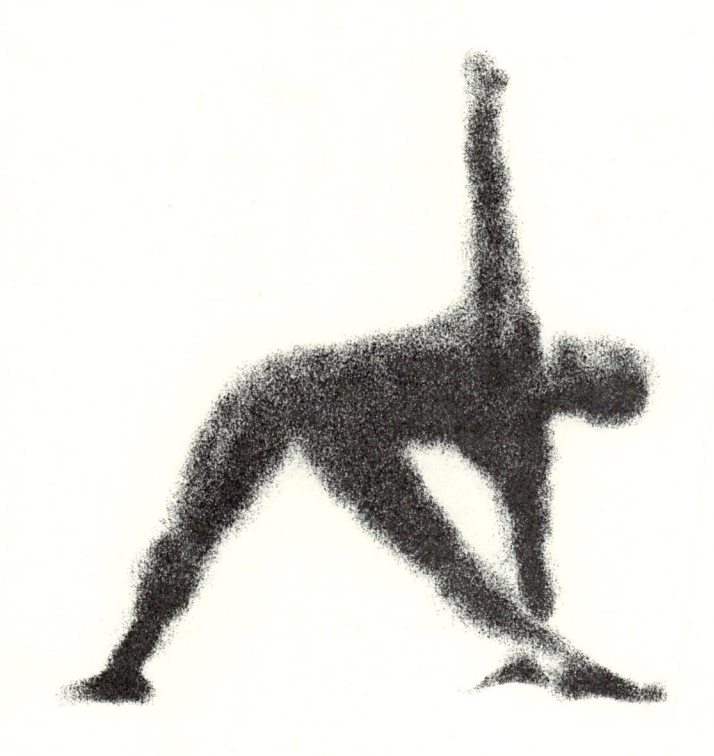

It is possible to see many intersecting triangles within this pose. But the foundation begins with a solid base and a firmly established rear leg. Any sense of hanging off the front hip joint indicates jammed energy rather than intersection.

Warrior 1 *(Virabhadrasana 1)*

Warrior 2 *(Virabhadrasana 2)*

Virabhadra is the name of a powerful hero in Hindu legend. All warrior poses cultivate the heroic strength that is required for union of body, mind, and spirit. It is worth noting that there is nothing about either of these poses that is particularly war-like: no weapons, no assault-ready stance. However, they do exemplify a focused readiness.

The warriors of yoga would seem to be ready for anything except attack on another. Both poses are balanced and poised. They are potent with a combination of physical strength and willingness to serve. The gaze is aimed and trained to see beyond and through what we accept as reality; the heart area is wide open and ready to serve a higher purpose; even the inner ears are balanced and open to hear the call of Spirit.

Once that call comes, the real battle will begin for most of us—the battle to believe what we heard; the struggle to stay aligned with our truth, even if it is not convenient or comfortable; the inner war with our own ego, which has its own very strict agenda; and the battle of facing fear and moving forward anyway even when we don't know what the answers are. There is no surrender (in the sense of backing down) in the warrior poses; rather there is an utter willingness to offer our strengths, whatever they may be, in full faith. That is the significance of the deeply bent knee: it is a sign of the ego's genuflection to Spirit's call.

These are warriors engaged in raising their own consciousness, not in forcing anyone else into compliance.

Energy Signature: Warrior 1

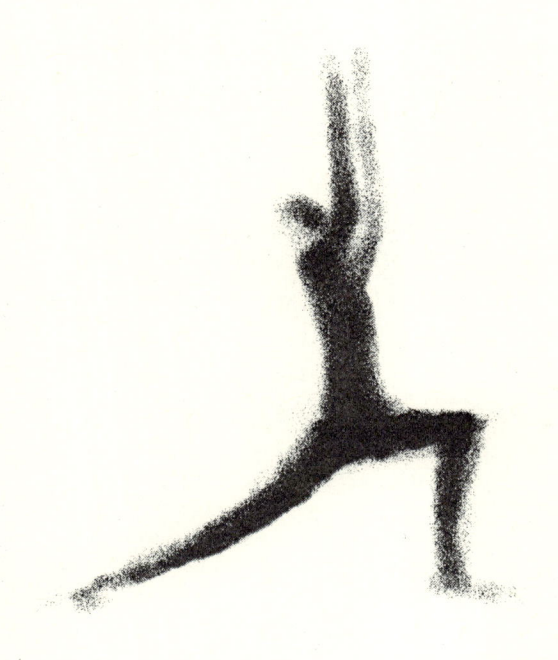

Warrior 1 and Warrior 2 are balanced, poised, and potent with a combination of physical strength and willingness to serve. The gaze is aimed and trained to see beyond and through what we accept as reality; the heart area is wide open and ready to embody a higher purpose; even the inner ears are balanced and open to hear the call of Spirit.

Energy Signature: Warrior 2

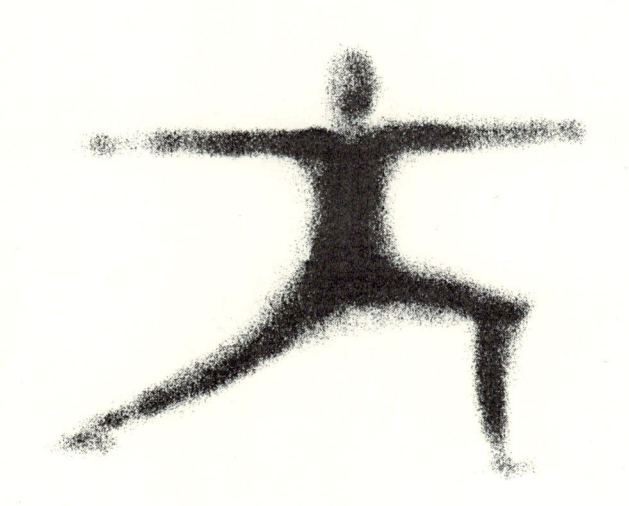

Chapter 3

Standing Balance Poses

Contemplation: Facing the Desire for Perfection

Standing balances offer a special set of challenges. They bring all of us—teachers and students, masters and beginners—face to face with our desire for perfection.

Even if you are unaware of your impulse for perfection in other poses, just watch what happens to you if you start to wobble in a balance pose. Suddenly you do not dare to breathe. There's a tightening of your chest muscles that cuts off all breathing. And what is that involuntary scrunching going on in your foot? Your toenails are digging into your yoga mat, and there's sudden tension around your eye sockets.

What's behind the desperation to stay balanced

long enough so that you please, please, please don't hop around like a demented bunny rabbit while everyone else in class is steady and poised in nice, neat, immovable rows? Where does that embarrassed feeling come from if you fall out of your perfect balance earlier than planned?

You don't need to be in a class to experience any of this. You could find yourself shamefaced, as if some far superior person were watching you fall, even when you're in the privacy of your own room.

Surprise! It's your ego looking right back at you. You have just met your rigid, unforgiving ego and its desire for control.

The standing balance poses provide useful instruction in humility, concentration, and self-forgiveness. They also teach us how to remain balanced and undistracted through the times of great change occurring all around us as we live and breathe.

Tree Pose (*Vrksasana*)

If you want to know how your own energy is affected by the behavior of other people in your life, just practice Tree Pose in a big class.

In Vrksasana, you are creating a whole new center of gravity for yourself. While you are earnestly trying to acclimatize and attune to center, other people may be swaying madly, like palms in a hurricane. This can be enough to bring your own balance to an ignominious end, even if the others survive and remain standing.

If some poor unfortunate soul beside you should happen to teeter just ever so briefly into your energy field, your peripheral vision or your sixth sense will register "invader," and you're a goner.

If only we could close our eyes. Well, we can. In a theoretical sense, it is possible to do Tree Pose with the eyes closed. Unfortunately, it's even harder with the eyes closed.

Besides the physical challenges of holding oneself in a stork-like position for any length of time, the bigger issue is that we can be distracted and taken off-center by the senses and by awareness of others. The tiniest little shift, the smallest of wobbles from "out there" is all it takes.

How can we be steady and comfortable without

allowing "their" movements to take us out of our own balance? Much as we might like to, we can never hope to control the movements of others. This applies equally to people and events in our work environments, current events, and home life, as well as yoga class. Sensitivity and awareness of others is a beautiful thing, but too much may deflect us from our own center.

This is why it is so important to cultivate the ability to see changes without necessarily being changed ourselves. True balance begins inside with being grounded or rooted. Tree Pose gives us the inside scoop on how to cultivate balance and equanimity with all that arises outside us.

Energy Signature: Tree Pose

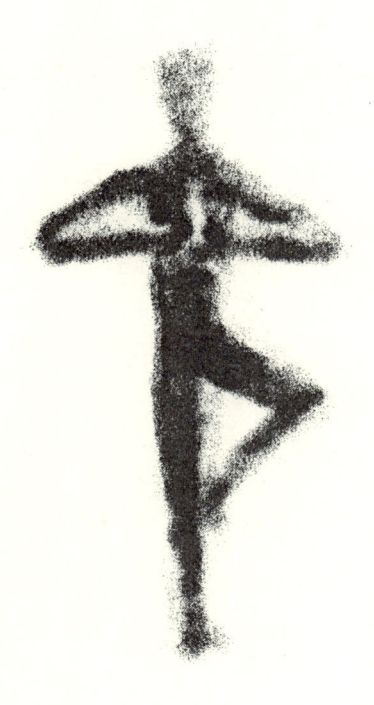

The energy signature of this pose is easily obtained by observing any tree. Practicing Tree Pose outdoors in front of an actual tree will teach you everything. Make sure that the raised foot is placed below or above the knee joint, not directly on the knee.

Balancing Warrior Pose—Warrior 3
(*Virabhadrasana III*)

Every time we walk, we are putting one foot in front of the other. Warrior 3 takes that everyday movement, exaggerates it, and then puts it under the microscope for examination.

What is it to take a step forward? When you think about it, it really is a leap of faith. Ask any toddler, poised on wobbly little legs about to take his or her first step out into the great big world.

To leave the security of standing with both feet planted on the ground takes faith. It also requires strength, concentration, and skill. While there may be nothing so very difficult for us about putting one foot in front of the other, there is in Warrior 3 the little matter of learning how to transfer our weight from two legs to one. Second, it's how to hold ourselves in the great chasm of the land of in-between. Third, it's how to raise one leg high without falling on our faces.

Warrior 3 magnifies the moment of transition and shows us what's inside it. Why do we want so much to get through this, to put our foot back down on the ground *now*? Could it be that we just want to get on to the next thing? We're busy people. We have things to do, places to go. Who wants to hang out in nothingness for any length of time? Aside from any physical challenge this pose presents, stillness is a fear-filled thing for most of us.

Try it. Be the pose and see what comes.

Energy Signature: Balancing Warrior

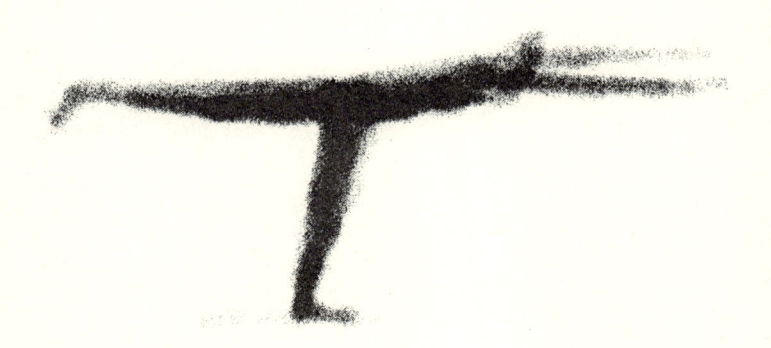

Grounded and firm through the core of the body, all else is "lift and lengthen."

Chapter 4

Belly-Lying Poses

Contemplation: Healing on All Levels

If you really need "proof" that the physical part of yoga practice (asana) is directly connected to the emotions, then practice belly-lying poses.

Belly-lying poses are known to be powerful healers. At the physical level, these poses can have a positive impact on some digestive disorders and certain bowel conditions. But there's more. Belly-lying poses can affect the emotional level, too.

There's a reason that we talk about "gut instinct" and "following our gut" when we're talking about absolute truth. Research has shown that we do have an enteric or gut brain. It has its own kind of intelligence.[1] If we lose touch with our gut instincts, we are lost indeed and wandering around in doubt and indecision.

Belly-lying poses put us right back in touch with our viscera and our inner truths. These are the poses that can help us get access to buried feelings, acknowledge them, and integrate them.

Practice any of the poses in this section as focus poses. You will likely want to leave the pose after a few breaths. Even four breaths can feel extreme. I can't tell you in advance what you're going to feel because for each person it will be different. But bring tissues and a journal–that would be my suggestion. Of course, this may not be your experience, but it certainly was mine.

There is no better feeling than that of being in harmony with yourself, and belly-lying poses can help with that. Whatever remains as undigested energy in you can be integrated and transformed through this practice. Who knows? You, too, may rediscover aspects of the self that have been forgotten.

---

[1] Michael D. Gershon M.D., The Second Brain, HarperCollins, 1998.

Energy Signature in Belly-Lying Poses

When practicing a belly-lying pose as a focus pose, you will need determination. But at a certain point, determination can cross the line into self-cruelty. You will need to find that fine balance and be very mindful not to cross the line.

Try not to just skim through the pose. Don't just give it a brief sketch. Fill the pose with real breathing, not the shallow little sips of breath that you can "cheat" with. While in the pose, let the breath be full, deep, and steady, letting it come right up to the collarbones. Let the pose develop staying power and character. Wait and watch attentively as it blossoms into fullness.

Deepening Your Experience with Sound

If you want to deepen your experience even further in belly-lying poses, allow yourself to vocalize. This will work in any pose but has some fairly immediate impact in the belly-lying poses.

It's good to have some privacy when you try this. You don't want the neighbors or the members of your household to be alarmed. It doesn't matter what sound you use, but a good one to get you started is "aaaaaaaaaah." Let the sound pour out of you until you run out of breath. Take another breath. If you can, keep letting the sound come from deeper and deeper inside you and just keep going until you feel empty (hollow). Rest, and then take up your pen and journal.

Sphinx Pose (*Sphinxasana*)

Before we could walk, we crawled. And before we could crawl, way back there in days that we can no longer remember, there came a moment when we lifted our heads up. Lying on our bellies, up went our heads, way up, like a brand-new periscope surfacing from the deep ocean of our beginnings.

For a baby, the head is heavy equipment. Being able to lift the head up and support it without flopping over is a big milestone in the life of a baby.

For the parent, it's a moment filled with wonder and magic. And yet we ourselves have no memory of that moment. It's as distant from us now as the stone Sphinx in the sands of Egypt. The only person who has memory of that miraculous event is the parent or caregiver, and that's only if they happen to be watching attentively. After that time, the miracle of it fades. Holding our heads upright becomes something we take for granted.

Sphinx Pose emulates a moment in our development that we cannot remember. When my children held their heads up for the first time, they were smiling. They were delighted. Babies make it look easy. Notice the effort that it takes as an adult to hold this position steadily for any length of time.

It is said that the Sphinx represents wisdom. If that is true, what is it that the Sphinx is seeing? Across all the years, across the expanse of time, what is it that you see or feel or know when holding Sphinx Pose as a pose of contemplation?

Energy Signature: Sphinx Pose

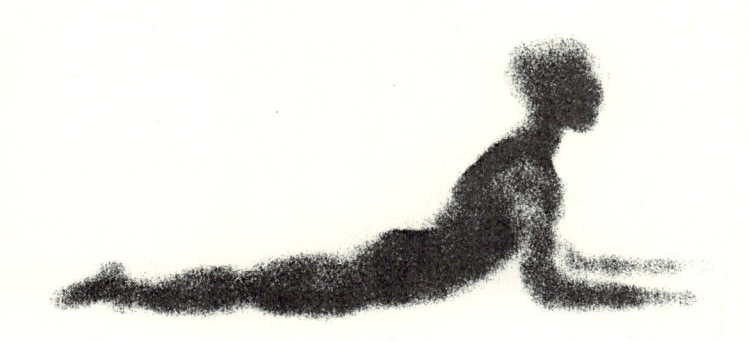

When my children held their heads up for the first time, they were smiling. They were delighted. Babies make it look easy. Notice the effort that it takes as an adult to hold this position steadily for any length of time.

Gently press more and more earthward through the front of the hips, the tops of the feet, and the arms and palms. As the downward energy connects to the earth, gently draw the heels of the hands toward your body and allow the upper body to find a sense of rising freedom.

Cobra Pose (*Bhujangasana*)

Snakes have been linked with mystical power through time and history to this day. Part of their mystery comes from the ability to slough off and shed their old skin—"off with the old, on with the new." Leaving it behind, they simply emerge as if born again into a new life.

People, too, speak of being reborn. This can happen in many ways, but all of the ways have to do with transformation. Your yoga practice, done with dedication and regularity and over a long period of time, practically guarantees you some kind of transformation. You may indeed reshape your body, but you may also find a new awareness or a new orientation that accompanies it.

When we can slip out of our old selves into new selves, we are leaving behind our old comfort zone to some extent. But first, we have to get comfortable in our skin and snuggle right up close to the edges of where we are now. Only then can we press ourselves forward into the new.

When holding this pose, it may be possible for you to sense the same kind of moving into yourself, pressing yourself right to your own borderlines, with everything engaged, alive, active, and alert. What is it that you need to let go of in order to be fully present?

Energy Signature: Cobra Pose

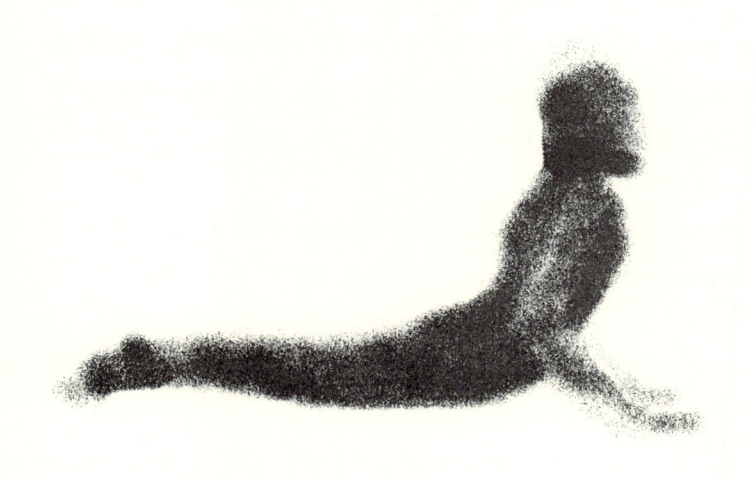

Note: It is a good idea to acquire a degree of comfort and stability in Sphinx Pose before attempting Cobra Pose as a focus posture.

It is said that the cobra doesn't use force at all to get into its most lifted and fearsome position; the strength comes from somewhere deep within. If you are using your arms to crank yourself into position, you are missing out on the very qualities this pose asks us to summon: flexibility, suppleness, strength, and timing.

Boat Pose (*Navasana*)

I have a soft spot in my heart for languages, even the languages I do not speak. Within the sounds of most languages I can find similarities to English. These similarities reinforce my belief that we are all connected, beyond time and place and culture. It's my pet theory, and the similarities between our languages demonstrate that for me very satisfactorily. The idea of interconnectedness permeates the very practice of yoga.

In what seems like a former life, I taught at a high school in Toronto where the students came from all over the world. Ninety-three languages other than English were spoken at home by the students. In an effort to find common ground at the beginning of the school year, I would ask the students in my classes to write the word for *mother* in their native language on the board. Soon the entire blackboard would be covered with thirty-five variations of the word *mom*. It was like discovering that the far-flung words were cousins; there were family resemblances that you couldn't miss, and the students were always surprised to see and hear these resemblances.

The name for Boat Pose in the Kripalu tradition is *Navasana*. The Sanskrit name is strikingly similar to English words such as *navy* and *navigate*, as well as to the French word for ship: *navire*. There may be other similarities in other languages as well. This is one other example of those mysterious little language clues that show how we might be more interconnected than we previously thought. So, perhaps in this pose, you can imagine yourself floating—not drifting or lost as a single boat, but moving steadily forward as part of a whole fleet, with your heart as your compass.

Energy Signature: Boat Pose

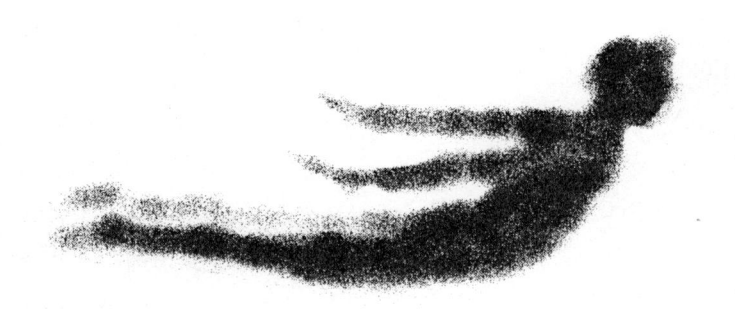

Imagine yourself buoyed and supported by calm waters, and see how the energy changes.

Bow Pose (*Dhanurasana*)

There are many legends about warriors and their mythic bows, blessed by the gods with supernatural ability and unerring aim. In these tales, the hero-warrior, protected by his magic bow, is capable of slaying many enemies and emerges victorious on the battlefield.

The goddess Artemis also carried a magic bow, which was given to her in her childhood. The twin sister of Apollo, Artemis had a preference for spending time in the forest with the wild creatures for her companions. She was proficient with the bow and arrow. According to legend,, she never used them to hurt anything. Her bow and arrows became the means to something ultimately more powerful. They became the symbolic link to perfect focus of her mental energies so that her thoughts and intentions would always manifest into reality.

When I was a student, Bow Pose cropped up frequently in our classes. Here's an entry from my journal from that time:

How long is forever? Forever is Bow Pose.

Bow Pose again today. I have an extreme aversion to this pose. I dread it. I hate it. However, I do not want to be the one to let go first. It would kill me to let go before anyone else in the class. And it kills me to hold on. I sweat, afraid even to breathe just in case my slippery hands might fly right off my ankles... body not in pain, exactly, but not "comfortable" either. This cannot be what Patanjali meant by "steady and comfortable." Agony is a good word.... My mind screaming "let me outta here!", "I can't do this!"... and then blam! Just like a cartoon, I pass through some kind of portal into an emotional awareness so huge that it really made me sit up mentally. I can only describe this as sitting up inside my mind. Now, where did this awareness come from?

I conclude that there was an element of grace in this. If it hadn't been for Bow Pose and the practice of reflection in my journal, I might never have known what my aversion was all about. Eventually, after I uncovered it and understood it, it passed, like a storm system passes over the coast. And it left me much stronger and much more focused.

Protracted holding of any pose, and, in my case, especially Bow Pose, can bring you rather speedily to your own dormant truth. I do like to warn students that this is a pose that can wake you up! Perhaps the fiercest enemies really are our own misguided thoughts, and therefore the perfect weapon may indeed be Bow Pose.

Energy Signature: Bow Pose

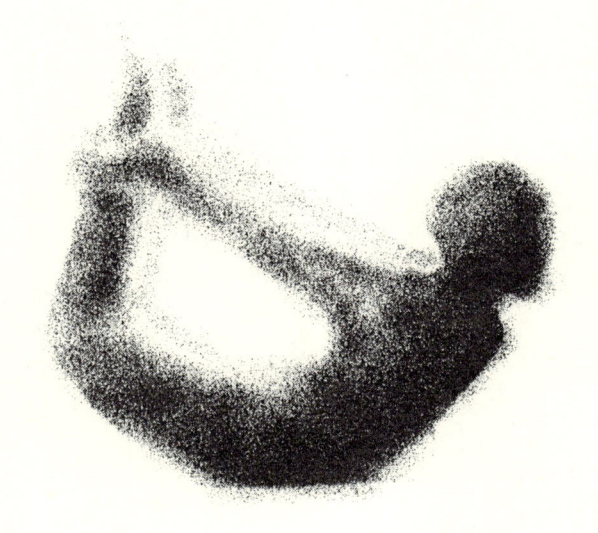

It's worth noting that the term is "draw" the bow, as opposed to pull, crank, or force. "Draw" your bow so that it is vibrant and taut without being wound too tightly. The heart must be light and lifted up in order for the pose to open up. This creates an unobstructed pathway from the gut brain to the heart and the mind. The breath is smooth and complete. If you cannot breathe, or if you are just sipping your breath, you have gone over the line—past focus and into brute strength.

Chapter 5

Three Poses from Hands and Knees
(Table Position)

Downward-Facing Dog Pose
(*Adho Mukha Svanasana*)

This pose has become an icon in North American yoga practice. Affectionately known as "Down Dog" it is often used as a transition pose in vinyasa practice. Also, possibly because of the popularity of Ashtanga yoga, Down Dog has become one of the most-favored and elite poses for all-over toning and strength.

Consequently, there are not many poses that have been so dissected in terms of correctness of technique, optimum musculature, and proper alignment. Open any book or go to any class, and there you will find copious refinements to occupy you as you enter, hold, and leave Down Dog.

Even after thirty years of practicing yoga, I can say that every Down Dog that I do is different in some way. This pose really represents to me how my own practice has evolved.

For a couple of years, I was obsessed with creating a perfectly elongated spine with a well-articulated dog tilt in the pelvis. Then my focus shifted to lifting the quads—I think this occupied me for a full year. Through the practice of Down Dog, I have discovered many interior landscapes, territories, and techniques. I have learned about the rotation of arm bones, I have strengthened my arms and legs, and I have learned how to release my thoracic spine toward my thighs. I have injured myself, too, in this pose from sheer overenthusiasm and what we could call overdoing it.

Despite its many benefits and refinements, Down Dog has an even bigger service to offer at this time. In an era when security and safety seem threatened, any pose that asks us to turn the world upside down and find stability is of real benefit in establishing a sense of inner security. The following exercise is an example.

Belly Awareness in Downward-Facing Dog

Come into the pose the best way you know how. Find the ground with your hands and feet. Find the sky with your tailbone. (It's absolutely okay to bend your knees if you need to.)

Now, forget about the rules of the pose. Make sure your body feels stable, but stop giving attention to whether your spine is lengthened fully or if your heels are touching the mat. Just for now, forget about perfecting the pose.

Just for now, concentrate on breathing. Breathe smoothly and steadily. Breathe in and out through the nose. Do not force the breath. It's nothing fancy—just full yogic breathing. If you must strive for something, strive to allow the breath to be deeply received by the body. Breathe as if your heart, hips, and shoulders just put out the welcome mat for the breath: *Welcome, Breath! Please come in.*

Once the breath is smooth and regular, notice how the body feels. Take a break if you need to, coming into Table Pose or Child's Pose. Just keep breathing smoothly. When you are ready, reenter Down Dog.

Your smooth, steady breathing established, begin to shift your awareness to the exhalation. Become more simpatico with your exhale than your inhale. Practice this way until you can feel the belly drawing inward toward the spine when you exhale. Once you feel the movement of your belly, keep your awareness there. Next time you exhale, gently press toward the earth with hands and feet and skyward with the tailbone. Keep breathing. Notice what changes and what moves, even the slightest, tiniest bit. Finally, lift the pelvic floor inward and upward, and hold the pose until you are ready to release.

Then come down smoothly into Table Pose and into Child's Pose. Rest here at least a full minute, longer if possible. Then journal about the experience.

Energy Signature: Downward-Facing Dog Pose

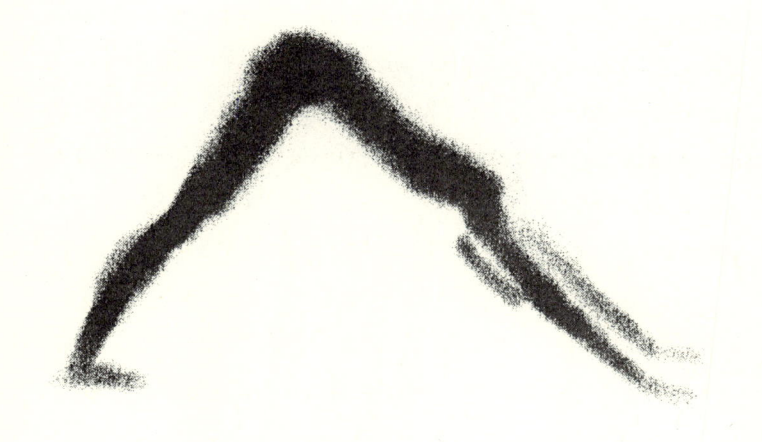

Pigeon Pose (*Kapotasana*)

It is said that the body mirrors the mind. A flexible mind equals a flexible body, and vice versa: an inflexible mind mirrors an inflexible body.

According to the theory, then, if you are especially strong-minded or if you keep an extra tight rein on your thoughts, you may have some problems with physical flexibility. On the other hand, oh-so-supple individuals who have no problem with flexibility may find that they are so "giving" that they get pushed around or bent out of shape by others.

It's just a theory. But Pigeon Pose is the perfect pose for considering our own unique blend of flexibility and strength. Too much of either quality will unbalance the energy of the pose.

In order to create steadiness and any degree of comfort in Pigeon Pose, there must be enough "give" in the hip, the knee, and the spine and pelvis. However, if there is too much give, we may end up with an injury, especially in the lower back.

Flexibility alone cannot sustain Pigeon Pose. Without strength, the pose can never lift itself into alertness and sweetness.

If there is an imbalance, what can you do to even the balance? Notice that if you want to force yourself into position, that might be a form of holding your thoughts too tightly right there. Sometimes, restriction can be related to a kind of mental resistance. The power of reflection can reveal this to you. Let the truth of yourself percolate to the surface as you hold the pose.

Energy Signature: Pigeon Pose

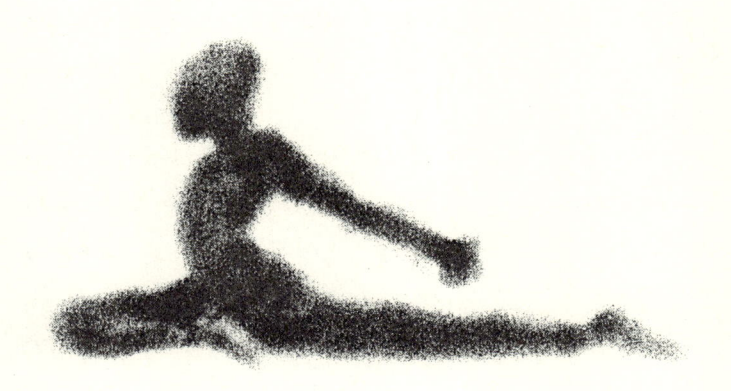

Pigeon Pose allows us to consider our own unique blend of flexibility and strength. Too much of either quality will unbalance the energy of the pose.

Child's Pose (*Garbasana*)

For little ones, this is a pose of comfort. It is the body-memory of the fetal position inside the mother's womb. The feet fold neatly underneath, and the bottom drops right down onto the heels. The head turns to one side, and they sleep.

For an adult, Child's Pose presents some major challenges. If we still had the soft bones and pliable bodies of a small child, we could settle quite naturally and easily into this pose. Adult joints that may have stiffened and body tissues that may have locked into patterns of resistance make it no simple matter to enjoy any degree of comfort in Child's Pose.

This is a pose that seems very simple. However, it will not respond to force, brute strength, or an aggressive attitude. You can vary the placement of the arms, but this is one pose for which there is no "progression" or advanced version. And yet, Garbasana has many levels, all of which look basically the same. It is by "being" the pose that you can discover the deeper levels of the pose.

At the physical level, Garbasana can remind us that, as adults, we may have lost some of our original flexibility. Inflexibility can manifest in other ways, too. Mentally, we can become toughened by life. Somehow we forget what it is to trust the process of life. If we are to live in the joy that is our birthright, we can come to this pose to be reminded again of what it is to trust life.

Garbasana is a healing pose for toughened or bruised spirits. The simplicity of the pose is possibly even more challenging than Headstand or Full Lotus. See what happens when you just rest here for awhile, practicing the five keywords: breathe, relax, feel, watch, and allow.

Energy Signature: Child's Pose

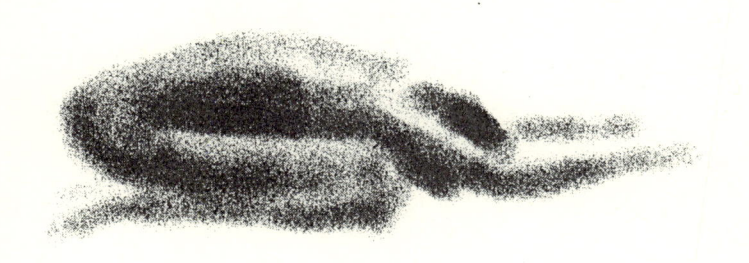

Garbasana is a healing pose for toughened or bruised spirits. As the body folds in upon itself and as the forehead rests on the mat, there is a great letting go for body and mind. The inner energy relaxes downward, the spine finds length, and the mind becomes still.

Note: There are many ways to support your body in this pose if needed. Do not hesitate to place a pillow in the fold of the knees or a small rolled towel under the fronts of the ankles if that's what you need.

Chapter 6

Forward Bends

Contemplation: The Symbolism of Forward Bends

Symbolically, the front of the body represents our awareness. In belly-lying poses, we lift our awareness up and out into the world. In forward bends, as the upper body lowers itself toward the lower body, we are bringing our awareness back toward the self.

There is a self-reflective element to forward bends. It's as if we were to bend over a stream or well to gaze at our own reflections in the water. Unfortunately, the approach is too often one of grit and sheer determination to "get there." As a teacher, I have witnessed much clenching of teeth, frowning of foreheads, straining, sweating, and just plain cheating to make forward bends happen.

Forward bends offer many benefits. For instance, they are soothing for the nervous system and calming for the mind. But you can see the problem. If the approach is one of force and strain, then surely soothing and calming cannot be the result. These are some of the easiest poses to injure yourself in.

It's a funny business, this business of self-reflection. We want it, but we don't want it to take too long. We hurtle through the mechanics of a forward bend as if the result must show up on the counter like a burger at a drive-through. We may be a fast-food culture, but self-awareness is not a quick fix. Think of a forward bend as a five-course meal at the best restaurant. There is much to enjoy on the way to dessert.

Hero Pose (*Virasana*)

When things start getting too intense, one reaction is to look for the nearest exit and flee immediately. The equal and opposite reaction is to lash out. It's known as the fight or flight response, and it comes up in yoga as well as in life.

What is intense in our day-to-day lives? Taking an exam is pretty intense; some people stay in the exam room not one second longer than the minimum required because of the intensity. Traffic jams can be intense precisely because you can't leave when you want to; when exit strategies are foiled, then aggressive behavior escalates. Listening to someone else's music blasting through your open windows in the summer brings up strong reactions, and so does walking into the middle of someone else's argument in a meeting. Any situation can take you right into your own fight or flight response.

What is it about intensity that causes us so much suffering? What exactly is it we want to get away from? These are two excellent questions to mull while holding Hero Pose. Because the nature of the stretch in this pose is so intense for most people, it's excellent for observing the mind and the body in the midst of intensity. There is an opportunity to appreciate the difference between actual pain and the richness of full sensation.

This is not a pose to force our way into. If the body isn't ready, it's just not ready. With practice, we build tolerance for intensity. We don't need to cut and run, nor do we need to create pain for ourselves. We can choose to face our experiences calmly. We can realize that there are other alternatives. We become more conscious of our responses.

Breathe. Relax. Feel. Watch. Allow.

Can you resist the temptation to flee and let yourself be present for your own "sound and light show"? Can you stay only if you are fighting it with your whole being? Or is there somewhere you can soften, even a little, and is there some peace that you can find in the midst of your intense experience?

Energy Signature: Hero Pose

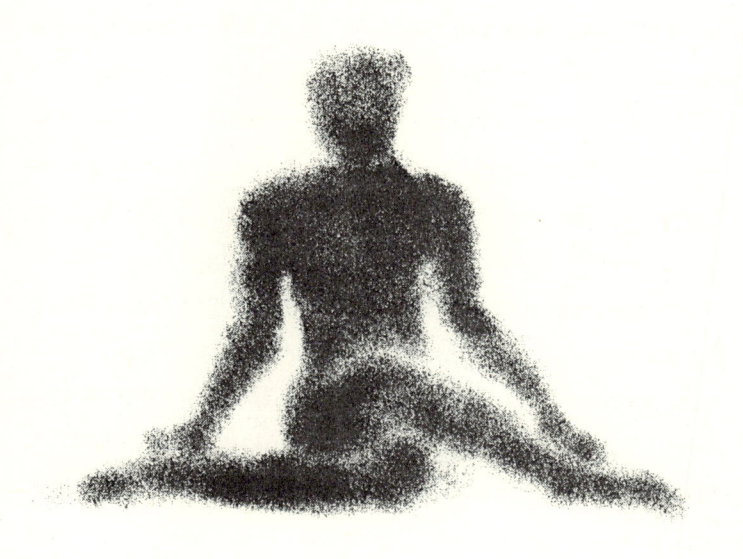

All forward bends begin with sitting well. Two elements of sitting well are that the sitting bones are grounded and balanced and the spine is elongated. *You may need to use a pillow or folded blanket under the hips to remove strain from the knees or to balance the hips.*

Hero Pose with Forward Bend

Once you are well seated, consider folding forward over the legs. Make sure that the fold is coming from the hips, not from the lower back. Stay balanced and grounded. Abdominal work is the unseen inner movement.

Head-to-Knee Pose (*Janu Sirsasana*)

The action in this pose brings the thinking part of the body (the head) toward the part of us that carries and supports us through all the pathways of our life (the legs).

More specifically, we are lowering the head toward the knee—the part of the leg that must bend if we are to move forward. It's almost like the brain is bowing to the knee.

If you have ever had a knee injury or knee tenderness, then you know how knees can indeed rule our lives. In that situation, we are forced to consider our knees before taking steps. We can't run off in any direction we choose. In fact, just walking seems miraculous after the knee has brought us to a standstill. When the knees are sore or tender, we need to be mindful of our steps; we are forced into restricting our movements, into choosing a path of least resistance. And we are forced into stillness. Anyone who has had a recent injury will know the frustration of this. But maybe, just maybe, there's a hidden gift: the underlying message of any injury may be that we need more stillness or some kind of course correction in our lives.

The body has its own intelligence. The body does speak its messages to those who will listen. There is a wonderful opportunity here in this pose for listening to the body instead of running it on autopilot from the head office (the mind).

Energy Signature: Head-to-Knee Pose

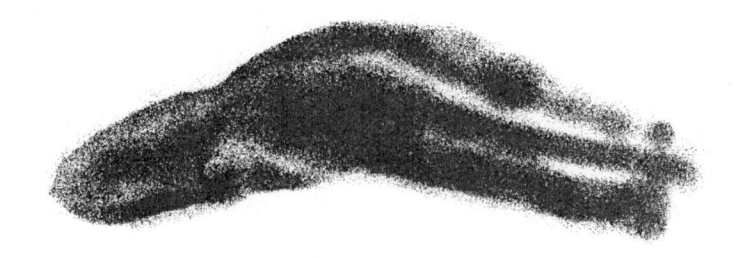

Some forward bends are done with a rounded spine, some with a straight spine. Head-to-Knee Pose is taught both ways. To keep yourself safe, make sure that the bend is coming from the hips, not from the lower back. The energy here feels more like folding a pair of pants over a hanger, not so much drooping forward over the edge like a flower from a hanging basket.

Seated Forward Bend (*Paschimottanasana*)

Using its Sanskrit name, we can liken this pose to the body's own version of sunset. *Paschima* translates as "western, last, final"; *uttana* means "highest, supreme, most excellent." The back body is traditionally known as the western body. In Paschimottanasana, the lower body represents the horizon, and the back or western body (the last part to face the sun) is folded toward the horizon.

A sunset can be wildly colorful, generous, splashy, and brilliant —and blazing like a glassmaker's furnace. When writing this book, I was in Costa Rica, where people would watch the sunset the way some folks go to concerts. People would gather on the beach or collect on their balconies, and all of us would watch the sun's spectacular finish to the day. But it was more than passive watching, as when watching TV. When the sun set at the beach, we were not just watching something— we were participating in a group experience.

During the day, the sun and its heat are more or less taken for granted. It was burning so bright and hard that finding shelter or shade was essential in the late afternoon. But by 5:30, the sun had transformed itself into a shimmering yellow disk low in the sky, which by 6:10 had vanished.

The Central American sunset gives us very useful guidelines about how this asana is to be entered: slowly enough to be gradual, releasing inexorably downward —not collapsing flat in an instant like an ironing board. Proceed slowly enough so that you are aware of what you are doing and what you are feeling.

If you were the sun in Costa Rica, you'd take forty minutes to complete this pose. I'm not suggesting that you must take forty minutes, but … what's the rush? Emulate the Central American sun: take your time, and be fully present in each moment.

Energy Signature: Seated Forward Bend

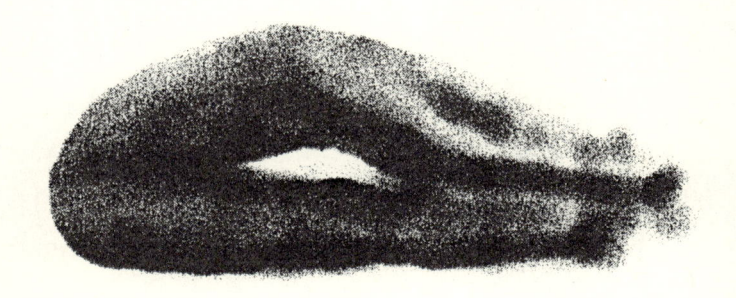

This is a good pose in which to practice enjoying the journey rather than the destination. Proceed slowly enough so that you are aware of what you are doing and what you are feeling.

Chapter 7

Twists

Contemplation: The Dark Side of Twists

There was a sassy little dance craze in the fifties called the Twist. It emphasized swinging one's hips from side to side while bending the knees deeply and leaning forward and backward. Athletic dancers could corkscrew their bodies right down to the floor and come smoothly back up again, twisting all the while. It was great fun and was actually fairly shocking in its day because of the hip action. However, overenthusiasm on the dance floor could easily result in spinal misalignment the next morning. The same is true in yoga twists.

In yoga, the power of twists is renowned. You can remind yourself of that power by watching the movie

Twister. Once the funnel cloud of concentrated energy gets going, it is an unstoppable force. It clears everything in its path. This may explain why it seems that more twisting poses are named after sages and yoga masters than poses in any other category of asana.

Whether on the dance floor, in the sky, or in yoga asana, there is a dark side to twists. Twists can be danger zones for vulnerable necks and lower backs. Sages must be discerning enough to perform spinal twists while respecting the body's limits and only when the spine and its surrounding environment have been warmed up and correctly prepared with sufficient preliminary poses.

When done with mindfulness, twists remind us to lead more from our true center instead of leading with the head. Theoretically, twists can take us right to the center of our power if we are sufficiently prepared.

Half-Lord of the Fishes Pose
(*Ardha Matsyendrasana*)

There are certain persons in this world who could be called headstrong. If it were a club, their motto would be "Just do it!" The headstrong are great at getting things done. They can overcome objections and crush all opposition in their path. They take some pride in being movers and doers.

The downside of being headstrong is that sometimes not a lot of listening goes on. When there is no listening, big mistakes can happen, which the headstrong may sincerely regret later. I should know because I belong to the club. I like to think that I have left most of that particular phase of my life behind me. I hope that I have learned my lessons and moved on.

Perhaps that's the sage's secret in this pose: the ability to look backward from where we are now with wisdom and equanimity.

It is definitely the perfect pose to teach the dangers of a headstrong approach. This is no pose on which to try the "just do it" philosophy. Twists usually come into the practice toward the end, after the body has become relatively warm, strengthened, and stable. The muscles of the lower back are like ropes in that they can be twisted gently; but if they are overtwisted, the result is a great big knot in the middle of the nice, smooth rope.

And it's really not about being able to twist your head behind you. A less headstrong, more harmonious approach would be to cultivate the twist gradually from the grounded sitting bones upward, using the stability of the sacrum and the strength of the abdominals. When the twisting action extends organically through the neck, that's where the true listening really comes in.

Energy Signature: Half-Lord of the Fishes Pose

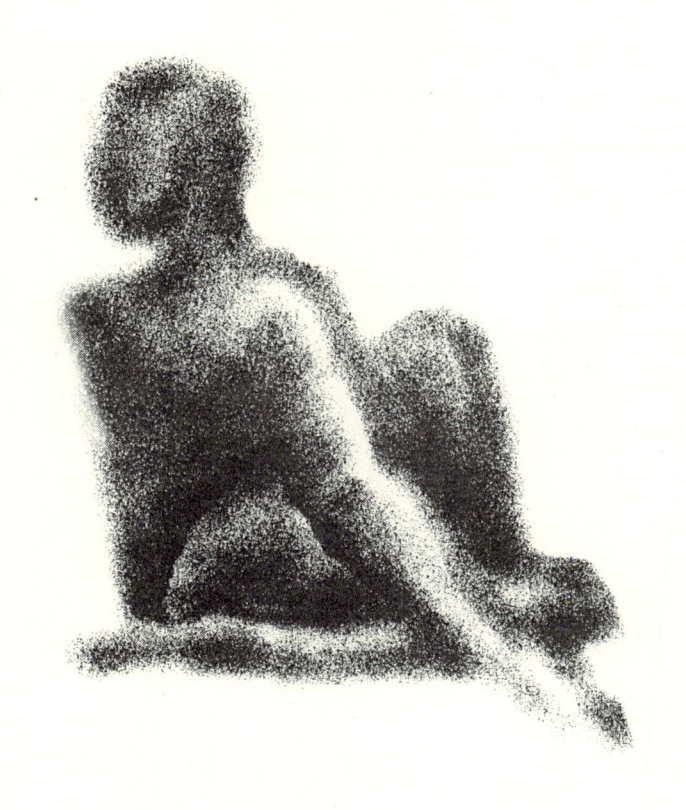

Ideally, the twisting action here will originate from deep inside the muscles of the belly, rather than from the muscles of the lower back. Before entering this or any twist, make sure the pelvis is level. Create and maintain a feeling of length in the spinal column first. Let the twist begin from your core muscles. Those with flexible bodies should beware of overtwisting.

Reclined Spinal Twist (*Supta Parivartanasana*)

Experiencing the Pause between Breaths

When used as a focus pose, Reclined Spinal Twist can be a beautiful concluding pose before Savasana in your practice. Create a spacious attitude inside your mind and body. Progressively give more of your body weight to the floor; and while doing that, focus on your breath. Let the breath become spacious, too. Allow the inhalation and exhalation to be equal in duration. You don't need to be militant about this; just start counting slowly to three (or whatever works for you) on the inhale, and then count to the same number on the exhale.

Notice any natural pause that may exist in between breaths. As your breath becomes regular, begin exploring the space that exists at the end of the exhale. Before you breathe in, let yourself rest or pause in that space for a little while, just as long as is comfortable for you. Keep yielding to gravity and resting in the space between the breaths. See how close to effortless you can be here. Then change sides and do the same thing on the other side.

Energy Signature: Reclined Spinal Twist

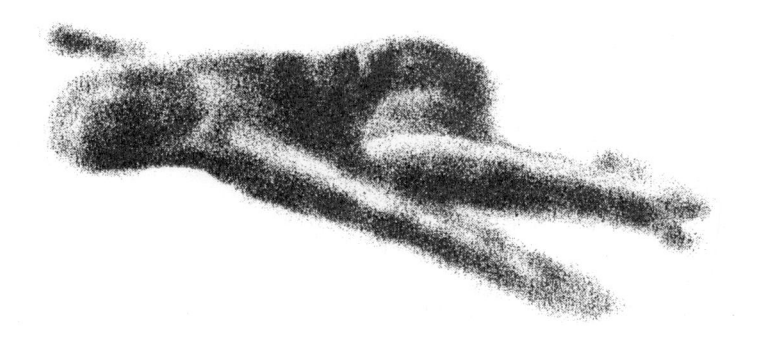

Yielding the body's weight to earth, cultivate spaciousness in the shoulders, neck, and breath. Gently allow the breath to slow down, and find a quality of gentle lengthening along the spine.

Chapter 8

Supine Poses

Contemplation: Working with Gravity

Supine poses allow the whole body to use the force of gravity instead of pushing or pulling against it. In relative safety, muscles that are usually exerting effort to keep us upright can relax and let bones fall into a natural, supported alignment. For instance, people with tight shoulders often find that the supine positions allow them to release the seemingly endless tension that resides there. Tight necks become softer and more spacious, and hips can balance themselves.

Supine poses remind us of the support of the earth underneath us. In the same way that life force comes to us from the earth through the soles of our feet, it can bypass the uptake system of feet and legs when we place the entire back body right down on the mat. Energy can flow more freely when it is not blocked by muscular tension.

The release of the poses in this section is especially sweet as it brings you to lying fully supine on the mat. Lying down is not "dead." It's just resting. It's temporary. And it will launch you right back into full form afterward.

Bridge Pose (*Setu Bandhasana*)

Bridges connect two far-flung points of geography that otherwise would be forever separated. In that sense, they give us access to geographical places that would not otherwise be available.

There are other kinds of bridges besides the ones that span rivers, lakes, and bays. For instance, the practice of yoga is a bridge to your own inner self. The Internet is an entire web of links and bridges that can take us virtually anywhere. In human relations, an outstretched hand, a kind word, an admiring glance, and a smile all qualify as bridges or connections among individuals.

If you look at the framework of Bridge Pose, you can see a human bridge. The yoga mat is like a map. On the map, the feet are in one place, while the head is far away in another county. And some days, the head (the thinking mind) and the feet (locomotion) *are* seemingly separate and disconnected—it's happened to all of us. But the journey to integration, no matter where you start the journey, involves crossing that bridge. And the only way to get across the bridge to the other side is right through the heart. The pose is a metaphor for human reintegration: oneness surely happens by uplifting and opening the heart. This is the same advice that the Dalai

Lama gave to North America a few years ago: open the heart.

Ultimately, it's a pose that can demonstrate to us that our own true nature is not far away; it is nearer than near.

Energy Signature: Bridge Pose

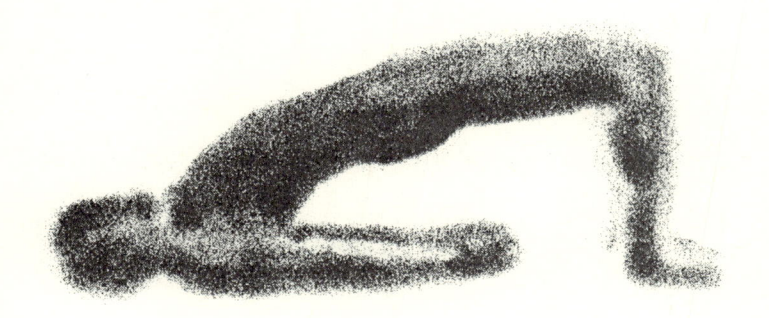

Pressing downward through the feet and legs allows the body to lighten and lift through the hips. Focused, earthbound arms and hands will result in a lifted quality through sternum and ribs. Engage the inner abdominals to protect against overarching the lower back. Bring the breath into the belly, and be the bridge. Small shifts will occur inside the pose. Notice where these occur.

You know you're using too much effort if your breathing is labored or shallow or if your jaw is clenched. Is that you frowning?

Fish Pose (*Matsyasana*)

This little pose can bring you swiftly and sweetly to the harbor of your own truth, the truth that swims just below the surface of everyday awareness. Fish Pose opens up the energy centers of the heart and the throat. If you are a person who clamps down tightly on your emotions or if you have trouble making yourself heard, Fish Pose can help you by clearing congested energy and guiding you to flow freely toward self-expression.

Come into the pose, and on an exhale, begin vocalizing an aaaaahh sound. Do this at least three times (more if you feel like it). Notice whether you feel any sensation or energy in the throat and neck. When you feel complete, release the pose. Lie still and witness the aftereffects. Stay attuned to yourself and note especially where you feel pulsations of energy.

Energy Signature: Fish Pose

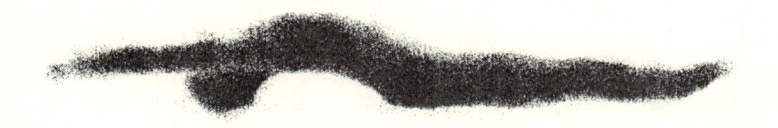

Grounded and pressing downward through sitting bones, legs, and heels, pressure is taken off the head and neck. The groundedness nourishes a lifted and open feeling through the chest and throat. The back of the head rests lightly on the mat.

Plow Pose (*Halasana*)

Plow Pose is named for the no-frills, traditional plow drawn by oxen, which makes the soil ready for planting. My ancestors probably used one back in the auld sod, and I certainly wished I had one the summer we moved into our new house. We had a fabulously large garden space behind our house. Armed with a hoe, a spade, and heavy-duty garden gloves, my husband and I set out with enthusiasm to turn the earth for our ambitious garden.

I made some discoveries during this project. My first discovery was that real earth does not equal triple mix. I was used to the light, easy soil you can pour from bags available at the garden center. What I discovered in our garden was the real, actual earth that had knotted itself into heavy, tenacious clumps. Some of them were earth all the way through, while some of them were really big stones covered in dirt. Hacking away with a hoe or spade for about thirty minutes would net a meager square of receptive earth, wickedly sore arms and back pain, and a bunch of rocks, all before even one tomato had been planted. Discovery number two was that rain was helpful because it rendered the clumps easier to hack apart, but it was also unhelpful because the earth became very slick and sticky, like a morass of raw clay. This has to be why wooden clogs were invented. (Just a theory.)

We did eventually plant our garden. Believe me, if we had possessed one of those old-fashioned plows and if we could have rounded up two oxen, we would have used them. I developed quite an appreciation for plows in general and Plow Pose in particular that summer.

It's helpful to have some imagination and a sense of humor to see things from the plow's point of view. Try it the next time you are in this pose. It's as if your feet are the handles of the plow, held by the farmer. Your neck is in the earth, and you are harnessed to two oxen. Wherever they go, that's where you are going. The farmer and the oxen can just walk over everything, but you (the plow) are going through it head (or neck) first.

The only way to survive, speaking from a plow's point of view, is fourfold: (1) you need to be in good repair, (2) you must be flexible enough to get through all the hard bits and clumps, (3) you must be strong enough to perform your task without giving up, since there's nowhere else you can go anyway, and (4) you absolutely have to trust that the farmer and the oxen know what they're doing. Until you are "unhooked," you are merely an instrument, part of a process that is bigger than you are.

When we come to those places in life that are hard, uncomfortable, and even stony, it may be more valuable to all concerned to stay put, see it through, and trust that you are being guided. Because of that, something new might grow.

Energy Signature: Plow Pose

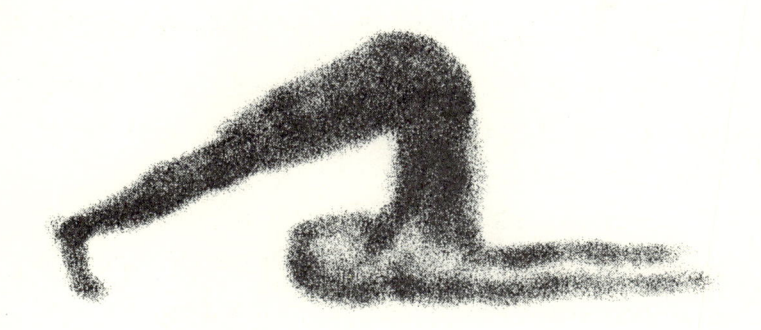

Become familiar and comfortable with Bridge Pose and Half Shoulderstand before practicing Plow Pose.

Although it's helpful to possess a flexible neck, much of the support here comes from the inner abdominals. Ideally, the body weight is supported externally by the arms and shoulders, not directly by the neck.

Let the neck be free. Find length and spaciousness inside. Be mindful. Cultivate equal parts of strength and surrender and allow the tops of the feet to rest on the floor or on a block.

Conclusion

Imagining yoga as a metaphorical baby in a basket sent downriver a long time ago, it is easy to understand that the basket has by now made a huge journey across worlds of time and space. This ancient practice of yoga has come from thousands of years ago and was transmitted across mountain ranges, continents, cultures, and oceans to land smack dab into the mainstream of North America. And the baby is growing up into a very wise being.

For those who believe this way, we are now living at the doorway of a great shift of human consciousness. Just around the corner, there are changes coming regarding what it is to be alive and what it means to be a human being. Several books have recently been published on this topic.

The presence in our midst of the ancient practice of yoga, designed to purify and enlighten us, is at the very least a happy coincidence. As a process, the transmission of yoga has been continuous and even miraculous at some points. For instance, who could have predicted that a swami named Vivekenanda would arrive from India in 1893, unknown and without a sponsor, only to be invited to speak days later at the World's Parliament of Religions in Chicago? His theme was "Harmony and peace, not dissension." Vivekenanda's remarks emphasized the underlying unity between all cultures and beliefs.

Swami Vivekenanda may have been the first, but he was not the last. How many among the yoga underground in the seventies could have forecast that over ten million North Americans would be familiar with yoga now? By May 2000, there had already been three National Yoga Conventions in the United States, and at present there are large yoga shows and yoga conventions held annually throughout North America.

Ladies and gentlemen, the baby in the basket has arrived and is growing up among us. At the threshold of change, we hold the gift of yoga in our hands, our hearts, and minds. Let us continue to nurture it and reflect upon our changes. As we nurture our yoga practice, we inevitably journey through change, coming closer and closer to the real self. It is my hope that the techniques and words offered in this book will help you evolve your practice as you yourself evolve, becoming more open to the changes in you and around you, and deepening your connection to your light and your truth.

About the Author

A Canadian, lifelong educator Fran Brunke, RYT, has been teaching yoga since 1998.

Born in Montreal, Quebec, bilingual by choice and educated to a master's level in education, Fran's background includes meeting the world at large as a flight attendant, raising a family or two, and teaching at a number of diverse schools in Toronto. She has been living and loving yoga for thirty years. Fran completed her yoga teacher certification at Kripalu Center in 1998. She teaches yoga classes and iRest workshops. She is on the faculty of the teacher training program at Blue Door Yoga Room in Woodbridge, Ontario. Having a special interest in the health benefits of yoga and travel, she has taught in a variety of locations throughout the United States, Central America, and the Caribbean. Fran lives and works in Woodbridge, and she escapes every winter to Costa Rica.

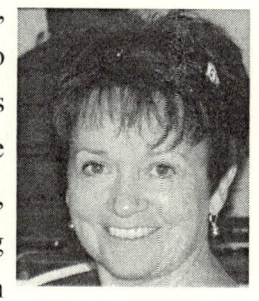